Mediterranean Diet Recipes

The Mediterranean Diet Cookbook is a Delicious
Beginners Guide To Losing Weight Naturally
The Mediterranean Way

(Simple to follow recipes)

Avent Lavoie

Published by Jason Thawne Publishing House

© Avent Lavoie

Mediterranean Diet Recipes: The Mediterranean Diet Cookbook is a Delicious Beginners Guide To Losing Weight Naturally The Mediterranean Way
(Simple to follow recipes)

All Rights Reserved

ISBN 978-1-989749-94-4

This document is geared towards providing exact and reliable information in regards to the topic and issue covered. The publication is sold with the idea that the publisher isn't required to render accounting, officially permitted, or otherwise, qualified services. If advice is necessary, legal or even professional, a practiced individual in the profession should be ordered.

- From a Declaration of Principles which was accepted and approved equally by a Committee of the American Bar Association and a Committee of Publishers and Associations.

In no way is it legal to reproduce, duplicate, or even transmit any part of this document in either electronic means or in printed format. Recording of this publication is strictly prohibited and any storage of this document isn't allowed unless with proper written permission from the publisher. All rights reserved.

The information provided herein is stated to be truthful and consistent, in that any liability, in terms of inattention or otherwise, by any usage or abuse of any policies, processes, or directions contained within is the solitary and also utter responsibility of the recipient reader. Under no circumstances will any legal responsibility or blame be held against the publisher for any reparation, damages, or monetary loss due to the information herein, either directly or indirectly.

Respective authors own all copyrights not held by the publisher.

The information herein is offered for just informational purposes solely, and is universal as so. The presentation of the information is without contract or any type of guarantee assurance.

The trademarks that are used are without any consent, and also the publication of the trademark is without permission or backing by the trademark owner. All trademarks and brands within this book are for clarifying purposes only and are the owned by the owners themselves, not affiliated with this document.

TABLE OF CONTENTS

Part 1 1

Introduction 2

Chapter I: Understanding The Mediterranean Diet 5

Chapter Ii: The History Of Mediterranean Diet As A Melting Pot Of Cuisines 11

Chapter Iii: Basic Principles Of A Mediterranean Diet 17

Chapter Iv: Exploring The Benefits Of Mediterranean Diet 22

Chapter V: How To Adopt A Healthy Mediterranean Diet . 27

Chapter Vi: Healthy Eating Using The Mediterranean Diet Pyramid As Guide 31

Chapter Vii: Mediterranean Sample Menu 37

Chapter Viii: Spicing Up Your Cooking With Mediterranean Diet Recipes 44

Herbed Clam Linguine 45

Bacon & Brie Omelet Wedges With Summer Salad 47

Greek Quesadillas 48

Mediterranean Couscous Salad 50

Mediterranean Chicken 52

Mediterranean Chicken-Pasta Salad 54

Easy Paella 55

Lemon Garlic Shrimp 57

Curried Salmon With Napa Salad 58

Baked Rock Cod Fillets With Olives And Pepper 60

Mediterranean Style Potatoes 61

Seared Mediterranean Tuna Steaks 63

Chicken Souvlaki 65

Simple Savory Mediterranean Chicken 67

Mediterranean Seabass With Tomato And Kalamata Olives
.... 68

Herbed Feta Dip 70

Scrambled Eggs, Toast, And Fruit 72

Granola With Fruit And Nuts 73

Omelet With Salmon And Asparagus 74

Vegetable Omelet 76

Conclusion 78

Part 2 79

Chapter 1 Lose The Weight And Live It Up The
Mediterranean Way 80

1. Munch On Vegetables All Throughout The Day. 84

2. Make Use Of Healthy Oils. 85

3. For Dessert, Eat Fruit. 85

4. Treat Yourself To Rice, Pasta, Whole Grain Bread, And
Other Grains. 86

7. Enjoy Your Food. 89

8. Drink Alcohol Moderately. 89

Chapter 2 Week 1: Let's Do This! 91

Gnocchi And Greens 92

Afternoon Snack 93

Morning Snack 95

Afternoon Snack	96
Day Three	97
Chapter 3 Week 2: We're Getting There!	105
Chapter 4 Tips And Tricks For Preparing Meals The Mediterranean Way	122
Conclusion	126
About The Author	126

Part 1

Introduction

This book explains the principles behind the famous Mediterranean Diet and explores the many health benefits people can derive from this healthy diet. It also explains how people can incorporate the Mediterranean Diet into their lifestyle.

This book is particularly helpful for people who are:

• Overweight and looking to shed a few pounds
• Exposed to the risks of heart diseases and want to lower cholesterol levels
• Looking to prevent certain cancers, obesity, and diabetes

At this point, you are probably wondering what makes this book different from other books that discuss popular diets.

First, the book explains the concept behind Mediterranean Diet in the most concise manner. It also explains its origin and gives a rundown of the diet's benefits when applied to a person's lifestyle.

Second, it provides the key components of Mediterranean Diet and shows how a person can incorporate the diet into everyday cooking.

Third, the book offers sample menus for breakfast, snacks, lunch, and dinner to help people get the utmost benefit from the Mediterranean Diet. The sample menus are especially helpful to working individuals who don't have the luxury of time to think about what to prepare for their families.

Finally, it contains several recipes that taste so good, you would forget these are actually dishes that conform to diet restrictions. The recipes are quick and easy to prepare, just right for busy individuals who want to lose weight but still eat delicious and nutritious meals.

Thanks again for downloading this book, I hope you enjoy it!

Chapter I: Understanding the Mediterranean Diet

Advancement in technology and the steady upsurge of the economy have led most people, to adopt a sedentary lifestyle. It doesn't help that eating processed foods have become the norm given that these foods are easily accessible. However, there's no denying the fact that these foods can greatly affect our health and well-being. These, and more, are the reasons why many strategies and methods are continuously being developed to promote a healthier lifestyle. Weight loss has become a trend, so much so that many people are encouraged to work hard to achieve the right body mass index for their weight and height with reference to age by subjecting themselves to one or more of the so-called popular diets. The Mediterranean Diet is one of these popular diets that experts highly recommend for weight loss.

The highly recommended Mediterranean diet is the contemporary expression of dietary patterns rooted in the histories and cultures of Italy, Greece, Spain, Morocco, and the other countries that share the Mediterranean Sea as a border.

This diet bears patterns handed down over the centuries. Its main characteristics are the extensive use of olive oil; high consumption of fruits and vegetables; the regulated intake of dairy products; diets that contain varying amounts of fish and seafood; limited consumption of red meat and meat products plus moderate wine consumption.

Recognition of the Benefits of Mediterranean Diet and Lifestyle

By the mid-1990's, the Mediterranean diet was praised as healthy, and its consumption rations were held up for the world to scrutinize. It was recognized as an Intangible Cultural Heritage of Italy, Spain,

Greece, and Morocco on November 17, 2010. However, long before this accolade was received, this diet was already recognized as healthy and beneficial.

It is to be understood, however, that not all countries in the Mediterranean can lay claim to using this diet as a part of daily living. In Northern Italy, olive oil is used for salads and dressings; lard and butter are used in cooking, In North Africa, the Muslim population prohibits wine, a staple (though taken in moderation) of Mediterranean diet. In the Middle East, rendered fat from sheep are customarily used.

Main Contents of Mediterranean Diet and Lifestyle

The Mediterranean diet stresses meals that are based mainly on plant foods, fresh fruits, olive oil, fish, and poultry. Zero to four eggs are the usual consumption per week, red meat is rarely eaten and wine, though consumed regularly by many, is limited to one or two glasses per day. Total fat in this diet is from 25% to 35% with saturated fat kept at 8% or less.

In addition to keeping high consumption of olive oil, legumes, unrefined cereals, and vegetables comprise most of the meals in the Mediterranean diet. Dairy products are eaten in moderation and even the choice of dairy products veers away from the extra creamy. As a whole, the Mediterranean diet is low on saturated fats, high on monounsaturated fats as well as fiber.

The good characteristics of the Mediterranean diet quite possible counteract the high salt content of many of the foods in that part of the world: olives, salt-cured cheeses, salted fish roe, anchovies, and capers.

Added to the Mediterranean diet, the Mediterranean lifestyle provides the necessary push for people who want to try the combination. They end up basking in the Mediterranean diet and lifestyle because of the resulting good health.

Components of the Mediterranean Lifestyle

The lifestyle includes a few simple daily must-dos, which are quite easy to comply with. One of the first things that this lifestyle dictates is the eating of small, frequent meals. The daily life of a person who is determined to follow the Mediterranean diet eats as many as six times a day.

The second thing that marks the Mediterranean lifestyle is very simple: daily exercise. The diet works well but needs to be complemented by regular, daily exercise. The other thing that is included in this lifestyle is making sure that the foods, the produce, are fresh and in season. Lastly, following a Mediterranean lifestyle means seeking balance and harmony in everything. In the Mediterranean, the original owners of the Mediterranean diet would have been physically fit not through daily exercise but because of their work (or labor) and their physically active lives.

More than a decade ago, studies showed that sticking to the Mediterranean diet and a healthful, physically active lifestyle lowered death rates by approximately 50%. This kind of endorsement can inspire many people to try the Mediterranean approach to eating and living.

Chapter II: The History of Mediterranean Diet as a Melting Pot of Cuisines

Many critiques will say that to use the term Mediterranean diet gives the impression that cuisine in that part of the world is homogenous. In reality, the foods and the cooking of the Mediterranean is a rich and amazingly varied collection of products, spices, methods, and traditions.

Impact of Geographical Realities on the History of Mediterranean Diet

In terms of culinary types, countries along the Mediterranean can roughly be divided into two major divisions: the Greek/Turkish/Arab cuisines of the eastern Mediterranean and Northern Africa, and the Spanish/Italian/Occitan cuisines of southwest Europe. Twenty-one nations on three different continents share the Mediterranean as a common border.

These culturally diverse countries are Algeria, Egypt, Libya, Morocco and Tunisia in Africa; Cyprus, Israel, Lebanon and Syria in Asia; Albania, Croatia, France, Slovenia, Bosnia and Herzegovina, Malta, Monaco, Greece, Italy, Montenegro, Spain and Turkey in Europe.

Early Influences in the History of Mediterranean Diet

Around the eighth century BC, the poet Homer wrote that the Phoenicians from the second millennium to the eighth century BC traded with Libya. He described Libya as a land rich in cattle, milk, cheese, salt, fish, game from the forests and timber. At this time Syria and Palestine were producing oil, legumes and beans along with fruits such as figs, apples, quinces, pomegranates, almonds, pistachio nuts, and dates. The Romans were also producing wine as early as 154 BC, and this, too, began to circulate as part of the Mediterranean diet except in the Muslim areas.

Wheat and other cereals were already consumed in the form of porridge and bread. To this day, there are earthenware bread ovens still being used in Morocco and Tunisia. Olive growing was very popular and so was the cultivation of fruit trees: pears, apples, figs, walnuts, hazelnuts, almonds, pistachio nuts, chestnuts. Dates seemed to be highly prized and were enshrined in coins and other artifacts. The Romans spread the cultivation of olives and grapes in all the lands they conquered. Therefore, it can be said that in the history of Mediterranean, the Romans created major changes in Mediterranean food patterns.

The Mediterranean diet naturally included bounty from the sea. The coastal areas enjoyed cuisine where fish and seafood were liberally used; they had access to mullet, bass, grouper, sea bream, red mullet, mackerel, sole, tuna, swordfish, prawns, lobsters.

While Homer made mention of Libya having cattle, elsewhere cattle were used as work animals instead of sources of food and milk. Instead, livestock leaned heavily toward the raising of sheep and goat. In particular, goat's milk and goat cheese were highly valued.

The Arab and Islamic Influence

The Arabs introduced new products and new farming methods in the Mediterranean. They brought or spread citrus, rice, sugar, pastas, chard, spinach, aubergine, okra, cauliflower, cucumber, and marrow. Apart from the bringing of new foods, food prohibitions were also introduced because of Islamic principles.

Areas devoted to vineyards were greatly diminished; the date palm flourished; figs, walnuts, pistachio nuts, and carobs that were ground as flour were reported at the beginning of the sixteenth century. Mention should also be made of the cultivation of aromatic, medicinal, and coloring plants such as cumin, caraway and aniseed, henna, saffron, oregano, myrtle, jasmine, roses, narcissi, water lilies, goldenrod, wallflowers, marjoram, violets, lilies, thyme, opium poppy and Indian hemp. The Arabs also popularized spices from the Far East: pepper, cloves, ginger, and nutmeg,

The Andalusians

Andalusians from Spain brought in plants from the New World – plants that were unknown in the Mediterranean. This included artichokes, different kinds of beans, spices, rice, tomatoes, peppers, maize, and potatoes. They also brought fruit juices, clarified butter, and other products that are still popular today.

All of the major influences in Mediterranean culinary history now make it even difficult to suggest that there is only one Mediterranean cooking. Mediterranean food is a mélange of cultures and pasts, one that offers experiences and flavors beyond imagination.

Chapter III: Basic Principles of a Mediterranean Diet

There are many varieties of Mediterranean diet but some characteristics hold true to all. These common characteristics can be said to shape the principles of this diet.

• The use of olive oil as the primary (if not the only) source of fat is a common denominator when reviewing the principles of Mediterranean diet. The use of other plant or animal-based fats is so minimal it is in some cases considered negligible.

- Eggs are eaten sparingly; often this is limited to a maximum of four times a week.

- Cream and butter are avoided; cheese, yogurt, and other dairy products are consumed in moderation.

- Fish, seafood and poultry and white meats are consumed at least two times a week. Red meat intake is limited to once or twice a month.

- Bread is usually consumed in its whole meal form.

- As a whole, the Mediterranean diet has a lower carbohydrate intake than regular diets and there seems to be a predilection for fruits and vegetables with a low glycemic index.

- Almonds and other nuts are consumed liberally.

- The Cretan version of the Mediterranean diet adds this rule: The main source of carbohydrates would be fresh fruits and vegetables, which are often served as the main dish of a meal rather than a side dish. Lamb, chicken and pork is consumed more in this version of the diet but olive oil remains the main source of fat.

- Spices and herbs are generally used to flavor foods.

- Red wine is taken in moderation at the rate of one glass per meal.

How the Principles of Mediterranean Diet Impact Health

Noticeable in the Mediterranean diet are the low consumption of animal fats and the regulation of dairy intake. The diet is good for cardiovascular health because of the type of fats utilized and the inclusion of generous helpings of vegetables. A major factor that spells benefits for the heart is the controlled eating of red eats. Small drinks of red wine and generous use of olive oil are two hallmarks of the Mediterranean diet. Most experts acknowledge both as heart healthy.

As a whole, the Mediterranean diet means less saturated fat – this is completely opposite to the regular food habits of highly developed countries such as the USA. It means allowing vegetables to occupy a large portion of the meal; using fish more than red meat as a source of protein and the removal of heavy sauces from food preparation.

Long-term adherence to the Mediterranean diet usually leads to weight loss, reduction of the risk of heart disease, lowering of cholesterol levels and cancer. The many benefits of the Mediterranean diet also include longevity, prevention of certain cancers, prevention of obesity and diabetes. Some advocates even go as far as adding that this diet improves brain function, keeps away depression, safeguards users from Alzheimer's Disease, wards off Parkinson's and relieves rheumatoid arthritis.

Experts have studied the Mediterranean diet and its alleged benefits for over fifty years starting with research conducted after WWII on which diets (by nationality) were healthiest. In most studies, the Mediterranean diet has consistently figured as one of the most, if not the most healthy. This makes it worth following especially now that delicious recipes have come up to support a trend that is hopefully here to stay.

Chapter IV: Exploring the Benefits of Mediterranean Diet

If you're determined to adopt a healthier diet and lifestyle, the Mediterranean diet is a perfect choice, as it allows you to eat well without feeling deprived. Why is that? Well, the diet includes such delicious menus and yet still provides what you need to be healthy. In fact, studies show that very few diet trends can outdo the benefits of a Mediterranean diet.

Key Components and Benefits of the Mediterranean Diet

The benefits of Mediterranean diet are a consequence of the way all its components work together. The diet has several key components around which each meal and each menu is built.

- Fruits, Vegetables, and Grains

Fruits, vegetables, pasta, and rice comprise a major portion of the diet of countries in the Mediterranean. In Greece, for example, the usual intake of fruits and vegetable rich in anti-oxidants comes up to an average of nine servings daily per individual while red meat consumption is minimal. This eating pattern serves to lower the level of LDL (low-density lipoprotein) oxidation and lessens the buildup of cholesterol deposits in arteries.

- Healthy Fats

Not enough can be said about the way the Mediterranean diet actually makes good fat available through different food preparations that include olive oil. This diet does not prohibit the use of fats, which are necessary for the body to function well. Instead, the diet provides the healthier choice of fats (the kind that contains linolenic acid, an omega-3 fatty acid) because of its heavy use of olive oil, canola oil, walnut and other nuts plus fish. The omega-3 fatty acids work in the body to lower triglycerides and are believed to provide the extra benefit of lessening inflammation. In turn, this anti-inflammatory effect helps to stabilize the lining of blood vessels, thereby indirectly preventing strokes.

- Wine in Healthy Quantities

Alcohol has always been a controversial topic in the medical field. Many doctors are reluctant to encourage the drinking of alcohol because of the possibility of abuse and because of possible negative effects on other aspects of health care. However, the typical Mediterranean attitude towards alcohol is one of healthy moderation. One of the benefits of Mediterranean diet and its adherence to consuming only the right amount of wine is reducing the risk of heart disease. Red wine reduces the blood's ability to clot, thereby acting in a way that is similar to aspirin. In addition, red wine contains anti-oxidants.

Incorporating the Mediterranean Diet into Your Own Cooking

You can do many things to start cooking the Mediterranean way so that you can reap the benefits of Mediterranean diet recipes. You can start by creating menus that include red meat only once or twice a month and filling up the rest of the days with fish and poultry instead.

You can also shift to baking, broiling, grilling, steaming, and boiling instead of frying. You will be surprised how good dishes cooked this way taste when you get hold of just the right recipes. Try loading up on vegetables – there are delicious many ways to prepare this when you go Mediterranean.

For snacks, try stocking up on fruits, dried fruits, and nuts. You can use these instead of the sweet cookies that are found in most kitchens. Switch to whole grain bread instead of white bread and take it easy with the dairy. Switch to skim milk if you can. If not, at least go for the low fat cartons instead of the ones that say full cream.

A major change you can adopt is to avoid cooking with butter and rich creamy sauces. Look for substitutes that call for olive oil and canola oil instead. While you are at it, read food labels carefully and avoid products that have hydrogenated or partially hydrogenated oils or saturated fats.

Chapter V: How to Adopt a Healthy Mediterranean Diet

The so-called Mediterranean diet is made up of foods that grow abundantly in countries in the Mediterranean. The coastline makes fish highly available and vegetables grow easily because of the mild weather. Olive growing is a livelihood in many of the countries in the area. As a result, olive oil is the common denominator of Mediterranean kitchens.

Bringing Mediterranean cuisine into your kitchen is not impossible as long as you have the following basic ingredients in your pantry.

1. *Olive oil* – an excellent source of monounsaturated fat, is an excellent source of monounsaturated fat, the "good" fat that actually controls LDL (bad cholesterol) level in the blood while boosting the HDL (good cholesterol). A first step in bringing the Mediterranean diet into your kitchen is to always have olive oil in your pantry and use it for salads or even fish.

2. *Fish* – loaded with omega-3 fatty acid, also helps increase HDL cholesterol. In the Mediterranean, grilling fish or sautéing it in olive oil is a standard way of preparing fish. A squeeze of lemon, some salt and pepper usually finish up the dish.

3. *Antioxidant-rich fruits* – part of the Mediterranean diet. Tomatoes are

especially popular in this region and many dishes are cooked in tomato sauce.

4. *Beans and vegetables* – staple components of the Mediterranean diet. Sautéed vegetables such as spinach and beans are easy to prepare; they appear regularly on the Italian table and should make their own appearance in yours as well.

5. *Pasta and whole grain breads* – frequent menu items for Mediterranean tables. Pasta is easy to prepare and light so it is common dinner fare.
6. *Nuts* – full of good fat in the same way that fish and olive oil are too. Walnuts and almonds typical snack foods because they are easy to prepare. Almonds are used to make pesto and are often used to garnish salads.

Apart from the ingredients that should be present in your pantry, you need to adopt some guidelines or methods as well. Again, these are neither difficult nor impossible to follow. In some cases, all a new convert needs to succeed in adopting a healthy Mediterranean diet is determination and a few recipe books.

1. Braise instead of deep fry. The less fat used as the food is prepared, the better it is for health.

2. Steam and boil whenever possible especially when vegetables are fresh. Plain steaming and boiling allows the plant to release its flavor without the distraction of other flavors.

3. Frequent, small meals are the order of the day. The ideal timetable for eating according to the Mediterranean is to take five to six small meals daily. This would include breakfast, lunch, dinner, and snacks taken in three-hour intervals.

4. Limit the consumption of dairy, red meat, caffeine, and refined sugar. This includes items such as doughnuts.

5. Regulate the consumption of alcohol to one or two small glasses daily.

6. Bring down the consumption of eggs to 3-4 pieces per week.

Chapter VI: Healthy Eating Using the Mediterranean Diet Pyramid as Guide

The Mediterranean diet has become recognized all over the world as an excellent pathway to good health. It is known as the eating pattern that allows the body to be relatively free from chronic disease and in recent years, research has shown that its beneficial effects extend to relieving depression.

What Is Depicted by the Mediterranean Diet?

The Mediterranean diet pyramid depicts the foods that are customary in the eating patterns of Crete, southern Italy and Greece. The extraordinary thing about this pyramid is that it might as well how people from these three Mediterranean areas ate during the 1960s. At that time, medical services in all three locations were limited and yet the rates of chronic diseases were among the lowest in the world and life expectancy was among the highest.

From a certain perspective, the diet illustrated in the pyramid was the diet of the poor people from the southern Mediterranean. It was dictated mainly by what was available and possibly affordable in the region at that time: fruits, vegetables, beans, healthy grains, fish, small amounts of dairy, nuts, fish, and moderate amounts of red wine. The

Mediterranean diet today is essentially what it used to be five decades ago. Ironically, the more lavish diet which could have replaced it is now known to lead to heart ailments, diabetes, obesity, and other health problems.

The Mediterranean Diet's Eating Patterns

More than half a century of research has gone into the study of the Mediterranean diet. A pyramid that attempts to demonstrate the Mediterranean eating patterns (relatively unchanged through the years) will show several salient features.

- There is an abundance of food from plant sources. These include fruits and vegetables, breads, potatoes, nuts, beans, seeds, and grains.

- The diet emphasizes the consumption of foods that are minimally processed. There is a preference for seasonally fresh and locally grown foods which optimizes the health-promoting micronutrient and antioxidant content of these foods.

- Olive oil is the principal source of fat which has not been replaced by other fats and oils such as butter and margarine.

- About 25 per cent to over 35 per cent of calories are from fat with saturated fat counting for no more than seven to eight per cent of calories.

- There is low to moderate consumption of cheese and yogurt with low-fat and non-fat versions preferred.

- There is low to moderate amounts of fish and poultry twice weekly and up to seven eggs per week including those used in cooking and baking.

- Fresh fruit is the typical daily dessert while sweets with a significant amount of sugar are consumed not more than a few times per week.

- Red meat is eaten only a few times per month and lean versions are preferable.

- There should be regular physical activity at a level which promotes a healthy weight, fitness and well-being.

- Wine, normally with meals, can be consumed in small amounts.

What the Mediterranean Diet Pyramid Illustrates

At the base of the pyramid would be daily physical activity. Following this would be a large section for bread, pasta, couscous, polenta, whole grains, and potatoes. The third level, divided into three parts, would be fruits, beans legumes and nuts then vegetables. Above this would be a section wholly occupied by olive oil.

These four levels comprise around 60 per cent of the pyramid, starting from the bottom. This shows that these items are the major components and the most frequently consumed foods in the diet. Above these, one will find cheese and yogurt then fish then poultry followed by eggs then sweets. The smallest part of the pyramid includes the apex and this is where you find meat.

The pyramid illustrates how eating patterns can be designed for longevity and good health. However, a good reminder to those who would follow this pyramid is that the very base of it is physical activity. Then, as every cook will tell you, Mediterranean cooking includes something that is not shown in the pyramid – herbs, spices, and seasonings. These add life and flavor to the healthy pyramid.

Chapter VII: Mediterranean Sample Menu

The Mediterranean diet is varied, rich, yet healthy. It is a source of so many delightful options leading to the creation of amazing meals. In fact, if you understand the key principles behind a Mediterranean diet sample menu, you will be able to design your own easily.

What a Mediterranean Diet Sample Menu will Show You

One look at a sample menu will inevitably lead you to the following pointers when you have your own culinary adventure:

- You should take advantage of what is in season in terms of fruits, vegetables, and nuts. The Mediterranean diet is heavy on antioxidants and unsaturated fats. These come from fruits and vegetables and as you study any Mediterranean sample menu, you will see the sense in taking what you can of the available produce.

- You must learn to switch ingredients in the recipes contained in any Mediterranean sample menu. Remove the foods you dislike but make sure you take into account the calories, sugar and fat content of the alternatives you pick. For example, you can exchange strawberries for peaches or chicken for fish but make sure you get equal value in the substitution.

- The Mediterranean diet is a healthy diet and any sample menu will show you that both coffee and tea are regulated along with the sugar that goes with them (1 to 2 teaspoons per day only). When wine is taken with meals, this is limited to one glass.

Every Meal Is Important

With the Mediterranean diet, no meals are to be skipped. Each one serves a purpose in keeping metabolism at optimum levels and ensuring that there is energy for a healthy life. The meals provided on this Mediterranean diet sample menu easily lend themselves to revisions. However, you can find all the products you need for every meal to plan your own menus in the Mediterranean Diet Foods Online Store.

1. Breakfast

Breakfast is the most important meal of the day and the body needs it to receive the essential nutrients it needs. Deprived of breakfast, the body's metabolism slows down. As a result, during the day you may feel cravings for salty or sweet things. Sometimes these cravings express themselves in a hankering for so-called comfort food. This indicates that the body has not received the energy source it needs. Two sample breakfasts would be:

- Yogurt 2% with rich in fiber cereals, fruit (three strawberries or one apple or one peach or a small handful of berries, etc.), and a small handful of raw nuts or natural dried fruits. Coffee or tea.

- Toast made from whole wheat bread, turkey ham and a slice of cheese, fresh orange juice or a glass of milk. Coffee or tea.

2. Snacks

With the Mediterranean diet, snacks full of protein and vitamins are necessary. Three hours after breakfast, the body needs some nourishment so that its metabolic rate does not slow down. A snack is also advised three hours after lunch. Here are two sample snacks:

- A handful of dried fruits, nuts, or a mixture of both.

- Two bran biscuits or crackers. Tea.

3. Lunch

Lunch is very crucial; skipping lunch will slow down metabolism and make you compensate at dinner by overeating. A lunch that has adequate protein and fiber will keep you going till dinner. Here are two sample lunches:

- Grilled fish, chicken, or beef with vegetables. Green salad with balsamic vinegar dressing (2 tablespoons).

- Lentil or white beans soup, Greek salad with olive oil (2 teaspoons) and feta cheese (30 grams).

4. Afternoon Snack

- Yogurt, 2 crackers

- One banana or one apple with cinnamon. Tea.

5. Dinner

Traditionally, dinner is the main meal in Mediterranean societies and the Mediterranean diet honors that. This meal should be well designed and should take care with the glycemic index of dishes so that the person eating it will be sustained until the next day.

- Green salad with chicken stripes, croutons, and dressing with olive oil, lemon juice, balsamic vinegar, and mustard (2 tablespoons).

- Pasta Neapolitan (sauce: 2 tablespoons), green salad with olive oil vinaigrette (2 tablespoons), a glass of red wine.

What Makes the Diet Work?

Take note that food intake is scheduled three hours apart. This is because it takes the body three hours to digest food. By keeping the three-hour interval, the body is consistently supplied with what it needs but it never gets to the point where it would store food and convert it into fat.

Chapter VIII: Spicing up Your Cooking with Mediterranean Diet Recipes

The Mediterranean diet is acknowledged as one of the healthiest eating regimens in the world. It is a diet rich in rich in nuts, fruits, vegetables, olive oil, and fish. It uses red meat sparingly and it combines this list of healthy ingredients with healthy ways of cooking. In addition to all this, however, Mediterranean diet recipes are very delicious in their simplicity.

Mediterranean diet recipes lean towards the use of legumes, nuts, seafood and fish rather than meat as the source of protein. Here are some Mediterranean diet recipes for you to sample, which were adapted or sourced from recipes posted on known websites. Proper attribution is given to each source at the end of the book. Once you try them, you will see why people who go on the Mediterranean diet enjoy both good health and fine food!

Herbed Clam Linguine

Ingredients:

3 quarts water

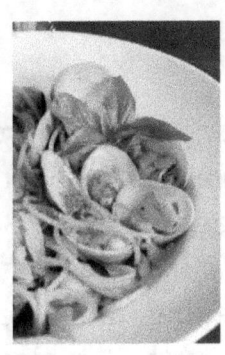

1 teaspoon salt
2 cans (6 1/2 ounces each) minced clams, drained and liquor reserved
1 package (8 ounces) linguine or spaghetti
1/4 cup butter or margarine
2 tablespoons chopped fresh parsley
1 tablespoon chopped fresh basil leaves or 1 1/2 teaspoons dried basil leaves
3/4 teaspoon chopped fresh thyme leaves or 1/4 teaspoon dried thyme leaves

1/8 teaspoon pepper
3 garlic cloves, finely chopped
1/2 cup whipping (heavy) cream
1/4 cup dry white wine or clam juice
1/4 cup grated Parmesan cheese

Procedure:

1. Heat water, salt and reserved clam liquor to boiling in 4-quart Dutch oven. Gradually add linguine. Boil uncovered 8 to 10 minutes, stirring occasionally, just until tender; drain. Return to Dutch oven; toss with 2 tablespoons of the butter.

2. Melt remaining 2 tablespoons butter in 2-quart saucepan over low heat. Stir in parsley, basil, thyme, pepper, garlic, and clams. Cook over low heat, stirring constantly, until clams are heated through. Stir in whipping cream and wine; heat through, stirring occasionally.

3. Pour sauce over linguine. Add Parmesan cheese; toss until evenly coated.

Bacon & Brie Omelet Wedges with Summer Salad

Ingredients:

2 tbsp olive oil
200g smoked lardons
6 eggs, lightly beaten
small bunch chives, snipped
100g brie, sliced
1 tsp red wine vinegar
1 tsp Dijon mustard
1 cucumber, halved, deseeded and sliced on the diagonal
200g radishes, quartered

Procedure:

1. Turn on the grill and heat 1 tsp of the oil in a small pan. Add the lardons and fry until crisp and golden. Drain on kitchen paper.
2. Heat 2 tsp of the oil in a non-stick frying pan. Mix the eggs, lardons, chives and some ground black pepper. Pour into the frying pan and cook over a low heat until semi-set, then lay the Brie on top. Grill until set and golden. Remove from the pan and cut into wedges just before serving.

3. Meanwhile, mix the remaining olive oil, vinegar, mustard and seasoning in a bowl. Toss in the cucumber and radishes, and serve alongside the omelet wedges.

Greek Quesadillas

Ingredients for Dipping Sauce:

2/3 cup plain yogurt
1 tablespoon chopped fresh dill weed

1 teaspoon extra-virgin olive oil
1 teaspoon lemon juice
1 clove garlic, finely chopped

Ingredients for Quesadillas:

1 cup crumbled feta cheese (4 oz)
1 cup shredded mozzarella cheese (4 oz)
1 small cucumber, peeled and diced (1 cup)
1 large tomato, finely chopped (1 cup)
1/2 cup chopped pitted kalamata olives
1/8 teaspoon salt
1/8 teaspoon pepper
1 package (11 oz) flour tortillas for burritos (set aside 8 pieces 8-inch tortillas for use)

Procedure:

1. In small bowl, mix yogurt, dill weed, oil, lemon juice and garlic; set aside. In large bowl, mix feta cheese, mozzarella cheese, cucumber, tomato, olives, salt and pepper.

2. Heat 12-inch nonstick skillet over medium heat. Sprinkle 1/2 cup cheese mixture onto half of each tortilla. Fold half of each tortilla (without toppings) over cheese mixture; gently press down with pancake turner.

3. Cook 3 quesadillas at a time in hot skillet about 2 minutes on each side, gently pressing down with pancake turner, until tortillas are light brown and crisp and cheese is melted. Remove from skillet; place on cutting board. Cut each quesadilla in half. Serve warm with yogurt mixture.

Mediterranean Couscous Salad

Ingredients:

1 cup chicken broth
3/4 cup uncooked couscous
1 cup cubed plum (Roma) tomatoes (3 medium)

1 cup cubed unpeeled cucumber (1 small)
1/2 cup halved pitted kalamata olives
1/4 cup chopped green onions (about 4 medium)
1/4 cup chopped fresh or 1 tablespoon dried dill weed
2 tablespoons lemon juice
2 tablespoons olive or vegetable oil
1/8 teaspoon salt
2 tablespoons crumbled feta cheese

Procedure:

1. In 2-quart saucepan, heat broth to boiling. Stir in couscous; remove from heat. Cover; let stand 5 minutes.

2. In large bowl, place tomatoes, cucumber, olives, onions, and dill weed. Stir in couscous.

3. In small bowl, beat lemon juice, oil and salt with wire whisk until well blended; pour over vegetable mixture and toss.

Cover; refrigerate 1 hour to blend flavors.

4. Just before serving, sprinkle with cheese.

Mediterranean Chicken

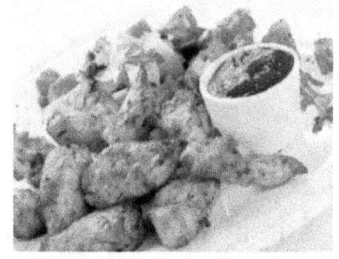

Ingredients:

4 thin sliced chicken cutlets (or chicken cutlets, scaloppini style)
1 tablespoon dried oregano
2 tablespoons olive oil
Salt and pepper
2 large garlic cloves, crushed
1 medium onion, diced

1 (15 ounce) can diced tomatoes, garlic and oregano style if you have it
1 (10 ounce) box parmesan couscous
Fresh parsley or oregano

Procedure:

1. Season chicken with salt, pepper and oregano, to taste. Add 1 tablespoon of olive oil to pan; when heated, add chicken cutlets, and cook until browned and cooked thoroughly. Remove from pan.

2. While pan is hot, add more olive oil if needed. When oil is warmed, add the crushed garlic and diced onions. Cook for about 5 minutes over medium heat. When onions are just about translucent, add the can of diced tomatoes (do not drain) and stir continuously. Cook for another 3-5 minutes.

3. While you are cooking your onions, prepare couscous as directed on the box.

4. When tomato mixture and couscous are done, plate your dish. Place couscous on serving dish. Place the chicken cutlets over couscous and top with tomato, onion mixture. This beautiful dish can be garnished with fresh oregano or parsley.

Mediterranean Chicken-Pasta Salad

Ingredients:

1 box basil pesto pasta salad mix
1/3 cup water
3 tablespoons olive oil
2 cups cut-up cooked chicken
1 cup cherry or grape tomatoes, halved
1 cup cucumber, coarsely chopped
4 oz crumbled feta cheese (1 cup)
1 can (2 1/4 oz) sliced ripe olives, drained

Procedure:

1. Cook pasta as directed on box. Meanwhile, in large bowl, stir together seasoning mix, cold water, and oil. Add chicken; let stand while pasta is cooking.

2. Drain pasta; rinse with cold water. Shake to drain well.

3. Stir drained pasta and remaining ingredients into chicken mixture. Refrigerate at least 1 hour before serving. Cover and refrigerate any remaining salad.

Easy Paella

Ingredients:

1 tablespoon extra-virgin olive oil
1/2 cup chopped onion
1/2 cup chopped red bell pepper

2 cloves garlic, minced
2 cups instant brown rice
1 1/3 cups low sodium chicken broth
1/2 teaspoon dried thyme
1/4 teaspoon salt
1/4 teaspoon freshly ground pepper
1 large pinch saffron
1 pound peeled and deveined raw shrimp (21-25 per pound)
1 cup frozen green peas, thawed
1 pound mussels, scrubbed well
1 cup squid rings
4 lemon wedges (optional)

Procedure:

1. Heat oil in a large skillet over medium heat. Add onion, bell pepper, garlic, and cook, stirring occasionally, until the vegetables are softened, about 3 minutes.

2. Add rice, broth, thyme, salt, pepper, and saffron and bring to a boil over

medium heat. Cover and cook for 5 minutes.

3. Stir in shrimp, squid, and peas. Place mussels on top of the rice in an even layer. Cover and continue cooking until the mussels have opened and the rice is tender, about 5 minutes more.

4. Remove from the heat and let rest, covered, until most of the liquid is absorbed, about 5 minutes. Serve with lemon wedges, if desired.

Lemon Garlic Shrimp

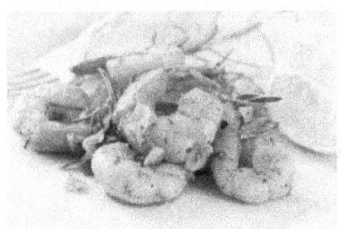

Ingredients:

3 tablespoons minced garlic
2 tablespoons extra-virgin olive oil

1/4 cup lemon juice
1/4 cup minced fresh parsley
1/2 teaspoon kosher salt
1/2 teaspoon pepper
1 1/4 pounds cooked shrimp

Procedure:

1. Place garlic and oil in a small skillet and cook over medium heat until fragrant, about 1 minute.

2. Add lemon juice, parsley, salt, and pepper. Toss with shrimp in a large bowl.

3. Chill until ready to serve.

Curried Salmon with Napa Salad

Ingredients for the fish:

4 salmon filets (6 ounces each)
Coarse salt and ground pepper

Ingredients for the Napa Salad:

1 pound Napa cabbage, thinly sliced crosswise
1 pound carrots, coarsely grated
1/2 cup fresh mint leaves
1/4 cup fresh lime juice, plus lime wedges for serving
2 tablespoons grapeseed oil or extra virgin olive oil

Procedure:

1. Combine cabbage, carrots, mint, lime juice, and oil; season with salt and pepper. Toss and chill.

2. Heat broiler with rack set 4 inches from heat. Place salmon on a foil-lined, rimmed baking sheet.

3. Rub salmon with curry, and season with salt and pepper.

4. Broil until just cooked through, 8 to 10 minutes.

Baked Rock Cod Fillets with Olives and Pepper

Ingredients:

3 large plum tomatoes, coarsely chopped
1 shallot, chopped
1 clove garlic, finely minced
1 1/2 teaspoons chopped fresh thyme
2 tablespoons olive oil
2 rock cod fillets (6 ounces each)
10 Kalamata olives or other brine-cured black olives, pitted, halved
Freshly ground pepper

Procedure:

1. Combine plum tomatoes, shallot, garlic, and chopped thyme in small bowl. Season with salt and pepper.

2. Cut one sheet of aluminum foil about and drizzle with one tablespoon of olive oil. Place fillets side by side in center of aluminum foil.

3. Top with tomato mixture. Sprinkle with olives. Drizzle fish with remaining one tablespoon of olive oil. Fold foil over, enclosing contents completely and crimping edges tightly to seal. Refrigerate for two hours.

4. Preheat oven to 450 degrees F. Place large baking sheet in oven and heat 10 minutes. Place foil packet on heated baking sheet. Bake until fish is opaque in center, about 15 to 20 minutes.

5. Remove from oven; let stand 5 minutes. Open foil packet over serving dish to catch juices.

Mediterranean Style Potatoes

Ingredients:

1/3 cup olive oil
1 1/3 cups water
2 cloves garlic, finely chopped
1/4 cup fresh lemon juice
1/2 teaspoon dried thyme
1/2 teaspoon dried rosemary
1/2 teaspoon salt
Ground black pepper (to enhance the taste)
6 potatoes, peeled and quartered

Procedure:

1. Heat the oven in advance to 350 degrees Fahrenheit or 175 degrees Centigrade.

2. Except for the potatoes, mix all wet and dry ingredients – olive oil, water, lemon juice, thyme, garlic, rosemary, salt and pepper – in a bowl.

3. Using a medium-sized baking dish, arrange the potatoes evenly at the

bottom, making sure you soak the potatoes by pouring the olive oil mixture you made in step number 2.

4. Cover the baking dish, and in the preheated oven, bake the potatoes for 1 1/2 to 2 hours. Make sure to turn the potatoes occasionally until tender but firm.

Seared Mediterranean Tuna Steaks

Ingredients:

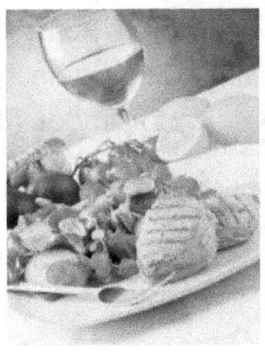

Cooking spray
4 pieces Yellowfin tuna steaks (about 3/4 inch thick)

1/2 teaspoon salt, divided
1/2 teaspoon ground coriander (optional)
1/8 teaspoon black pepper
1 1/2 cups chopped seeded tomato
1/4 cup chopped green onions
3 tablespoons chopped fresh parsley
1 tablespoon capers, drained
1 tablespoon extra virgin olive oil
1 tablespoon lemon juice
1/2 teaspoon minced garlic
12 chopped pitted Kalamata olives

Procedure:

1. Over medium-high heat, place a large nonstick skillet. Sprinkle fish with 1/4 teaspoon salt, coriander (if using), and pepper.

2. Make sure to coat the pan with cooking spray.

3. Add the fish to the pan and cook for 4 minutes on each side or until you reach the degree of doneness you desire.

4. While fish cooks, combine remaining 1/4 teaspoon salt, tomato, and remaining ingredients. Serve hot with the tomato mixture over the tuna.

Chicken Souvlaki

Ingredients:

1/2 cup (2 ounces) crumbled feta cheese
1/2 cup plain Greek-style yogurt (low fat is fine too)
2 teaspoons chopped fresh dill
1 tablespoon extra virgin olive oil, divided
1 1/4 teaspoons minced garlic, divided
1/2 teaspoon dried oregano
2 cups sliced boneless chicken breast, roasted and skinless
4 (6-inch) pitas, cut into half
a cup of shredded iceberg lettuce
1/2 cup chopped peeled cucumber
1/2 cup chopped plum tomato
1/4 cup thinly sliced red onion
1 tablespoon chopped parsley

Procedure:

1. In a small bowl, combine feta cheese, 1 teaspoon oil, dill, parsley, yogurt, and 1/4 teaspoon garlic. Mix very well.

2. Over medium-high fire, heat 2 teaspoons of olive oil in a large skillet.

3. Add 1 teaspoon of garlic and oregano to pan; sauté for 20 to 30 seconds.

4. Add chicken and cook for 2 minutes or until thoroughly heated.

5. Scoop about 1/4 cup of the chicken mixture and place onto each pita half. Top with about 2 tablespoons of the yogurt mixture. Add in 2 tablespoons shredded lettuce, a tablespoon of cucumber, and a tablespoon of tomato.

6. For the onions, make sure you divide these evenly among the eight pita halves.

Simple Savory Mediterranean Chicken

Ingredients:

4 boneless, skinless chicken breasts
1 medium onion, sliced
1 sweet red bell pepper, sliced
3 cloves garlic, chopped
1/4 cup sun-dried tomato, chopped
5 pieces black olives, sliced
1 to 2 teaspoons minced parsley
1 chicken bouillon cube, dissolved in 8 oz. water
Fresh ground black pepper
1 tsp garlic powder
4 servings of any small pasta
2 Tbs olive oil

Procedure:

1. Cut chicken breasts into small pieces, about 1" thick.

2. Mix garlic powder, ground black pepper and sprinkle over chicken pieces.

3. Put olive oil in sauté pan cook chicken pieces over med/high heat for approximately 5 minutes, turning chicken occasionally.

4. Add pepper, onions, garlic, sun dried tomatoes and parsley.

5. Sauté over medium heat for 5 minutes, being careful not to burn the garlic.

6. Add the chicken broth and bring to a simmer. Turn the heat to low, cover & simmer for 15 minutes or until chicken is cooked through.

7. Serve over small pasta done al dente.

Mediterranean Seabass with Tomato and Kalamata Olives

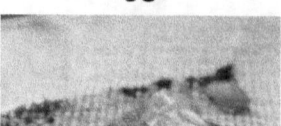

Ingredients:

1 tablespoon extra-virgin olive oil
3 cloves garlic, minced
1 (28-ounce) can crushed tomatoes
1/3 cup pitted kalamata olives, coarsely chopped
1 tablespoon capers
1 teaspoon dried oregano
Sea salt
Freshly ground pepper
4 Mediterranean seabass fillets (about 4 ounces each)

Procedure:

1. Heat the oil in a large skillet. Sauté garlic cloves then add the crushed tomatoes and bring to a simmer.

2. Meanwhile, slice the olives, pit them, and chop them roughly. Add olives to the sauce along with capers and oregano.

3. Add salt and pepper to taste; adjust the heat and simmer for 15 minutes.

4. Slip the fillets into the sauce, and make sure the fillets are covered with the sauce.

5. Cover and simmer until cooked through, about 15 minutes.

Herbed Feta Dip

Ingredients:

6 ounces feta
1/2 cup finely chopped fresh flat-leaf parsley
1/4 cup finely chopped fresh mint
2 tablespoons finely chopped fresh dill, plus torn sprigs for serving

Kosher salt and freshly ground black pepper
Olive oil

Procedure:

Blend feta and a splash of water in a food processor. Transfer to a medium bowl and mix in parsley, mint, and chopped dill; season with salt and pepper. Drizzle with oil and top with dill sprigs.

Healthy Options for a Mediterranean Diet Breakfast

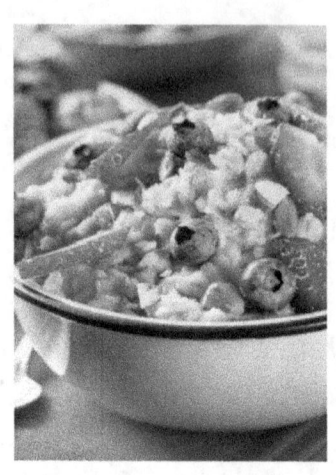

Scrambled Eggs, Toast, and Fruit

One of the simplest things to put together for breakfast is scrambled eggs, toast, and fruit. To convert the usual combination into a Mediterranean diet breakfast, simply use whole-wheat toast instead of white bread. This should remain unbuttered – butter is not used in the Mediterranean diet. Provide a full serving of fruit with this meal and use a nonstick pan for grease free scrambled eggs. Use salt, pepper, and a small amount of low fat or non-fat milk to make your scrambled eggs.

Granola with Fruit and Nuts

Breakfast on the run happens to everyone at one time or another. The nice thing about this breakfast is it takes very little time to prepare.

Ingredients:

1/2 cup low fat granola
1/2 cup low fat or fat free milk
1/4 banana, sliced and peeled
1/4 medium apple, cored, peeled and diced
1 teaspoon walnuts, chopped

Procedure:

Simply mix granola and milk in a bowl then top with the fruits. You can use any fruit you like but the best choice would be fruits in season.

Omelet with Salmon and Asparagus

This dish is so good you can actually have it for any meal during the day but it is a nice breakfast treat so go ahead and enjoy it. If you prefer any other type of fish, do substitute.

Ingredients:

4 ounces raw salmon cut into fine strips and pan grilled
1/2 teaspoon canola oil
2 tablespoons onion, diced
2 asparagus spears, steamed
1/4 teaspoon lemon juice
2 eggs (organic is preferable)
1 teaspoon low fat milk
1/2 tablespoon parsley
Salt, pepper, dill, and chives to taste

Procedure:

1. Use a nonstick skillet. Add the oil over medium heat and sauté onions for two to three minutes or until translucent.

2. Add the asparagus, garlic and lemon juice. Sauté for another two minutes.

3. In a separate bowl, beat the milk, eggs, parsley, and season with salt, pepper, dill, and chives to taste. Add the eggs to the vegetable mixture and cook for one minute.

4. Add the salmon to the mixture and reduce heat to low. Allow eggs to cook for two to three minutes the fold the omelet in half.

5. Cook for one additional minute.

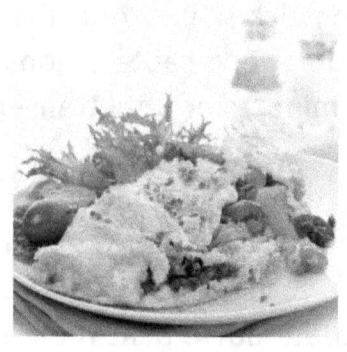

Vegetable Omelet

Sauté finely chopped green onions, diced red peppers, sliced mushrooms, and peas very quickly in a little olive oil. Season veggies with salt and pepper. Pour two large eggs, beaten into the vegetable mix and allow to set. Flip over and divide into four wedges when you serve.

It is easy to prepare a Mediterranean diet breakfast if you keep in mind the basic dietary principles of this diet. Once you get to know these principles, you can really have everything because all you need to do is to take the recipe for any meal and convert! That's why nobody on this diet feels deprived.

Conclusion

Thank you again for downloading this book!

I hope everything you have learned about Mediterranean Diet from this book will give you the inspiration you need to resort to a healthier lifestyle.

The next step is to select the recipes you would like to try, and start shopping for the ingredients. By now, you have probably noticed that most of the ingredients in the given recipes are quite simple and easy to find in your local supermarket. Once you have your ingredients, set aside an afternoon for cooking your selected recipes. The best thing about these recipes is that you can do all the cooking in one session and just refrigerate the leftovers for reheating later. Just make sure you cook a large enough batch since the rest of your family will likely want to try to some.

Part 2

Chapter 1 Lose the Weight and Live It Up the Mediterranean Way

Following the Mediterranean diet plan may be your best bet if you want to effectively lose weight and live a healthier, longer life. This diet plan is based on what the Italians and Greeks used to eat in the 60s. Studies have shown that they appeared healthier than Americans and were less likely to have killer diseases. These people were found to practice healthy eating basics while flavoring their dishes with olive oil as well as having some red wine.

Mediterranean Diet Benefits

Studies have shown that the heart disease risk of people following the traditional Mediterranean diet is reduced. Researchers have linked the diet plan with reduced level of oxidized LDL (low-density lipoprotein) cholesterol, which is referred to as "bad" cholesterol because of its likelihood to become deposited in the arteries.

In a meta-analysis study of over one million and five hundred thousand healthy individuals, it was demonstrated that adhering to the Mediterranean diet plan is linked to a lower risk of mortality due to cardiovascular problems and even overall mortality. Moreover, the Mediterranean diet may also play a role in lower incidence of cancer, Parkinson's disease and Alzheimer's disease. It was also found that women who followed the Mediterranean diet plan might also reduce their risk of having breast cancer.

Mediterranean Diet Basics

Eat the following foods

1. Regularly

- Fruits and vegetables – bananas, pears, grapes, figs, peaches, apples, oranges, strawberries, dates melons as well as

broccoli, spinach, cauliflower, Brussels sprouts, tomatoes, kale, onions, carrots and cucumbers
- Legumes, seeds and nuts – peas, lentils, peanuts, beans, pulses and chickpeas as well as walnuts, hazelnuts, sunflower seeds, almonds, Macadamia nuts, cashews and pumpkin seeds
- Breads and pasts (whole grain)
- Whole grains and tubers – whole oats, rye, corn, whole wheat, brown rice, barley and buckwheat as well as potatoes, turnips, sweet potatoes and yams
- Fish and seafood – salmon, trout, mackerel, sardines and tuna as well as shrimp, clams, mussels, oysters and crab
- Healthy fats - olive oil (extra virgin) avocado oil as well as olives and avocado
- Herbs and spices – garlic, mint, sage, cinnamon, basil, rosemary, nutmeg and pepper

2. In moderation

- Eggs and poultry – chicken eggs, duck

eggs and quail eggs as well as chicken meat, turkey meat and duck meat
- Dairy – cheese, plain yogurt and Greek yogurt

3. Rarely

- Red meat

Avoid the following unhealthy foods

1. Highly-processed foods

- "Low-fat"foods
- "Diet"foods

2. Refined oils

- Canola oil
- Soybean oil
- Cottonseeds oil

3. Processed meat

- Hot dogs
- Sausages

4. Refined grains

- Refined wheat pasta
- White bread

5. Trans fats

- Found in various processed foods like

margarine
6. Added sugar

- Table sugar
- Candies
- Soda
- Ice cream

Mediterranean Diet Tips

1. Munch on vegetables all throughout the day.

The truth is that most people do not eat enough vegetables. Strive to consume three to eight servings daily. Know that one serving size of veggies is equal to one-half to two cups. Choose the kinds that come in a wide array of colors to ensure getting a range of vitamins and antioxidants. You can have spinach with your favorite Cheddar omelet for breakfast, tuck into a big bowl of veggie soup for lunch, and sit down to a plate of roasted carrots with some green salad at dinnertime. By the way, eating green salads lets you have several vegetable servings in one go, so make sure to have one every day.

2. Make use of healthy oils.

Do away with margarine and butter (loaded with unsaturated fats that may be responsible for increased heart disease risk). You can use olive oil for all of your cooking and baking needs. Olive oil is a rich source of monounsaturated fats that are known to be good for your heart. Mix high-quality olive oil (extra virgin) with balsamic vinegar to create a deliciously healthy dip that will be a great substitute for butter. You can also make use of walnut oil and other plant-based oils that also contain high levels of heart-healthy omega-3s and monounsaturated fats.

3. For dessert, eat fruit.

Fresh fruits, which contain high levels of antioxidants, fiber and vitamin C, are your best bet if you want to satisfy your cravings for sweets in a healthy way. You may sprinkle a bit of brown sugar on a bowl of grapefruit or drizzle a teaspoon of honey on several pear slices to help you eat more fruit. Make sure to always stock up on fresh fruit at home and at work. Keep them visible to make it easy for you to grab them whenever you feel the munchies coming on.

4. Treat yourself to rice, pasta, whole grain bread, and other grains.

Have fun experimenting with whole grains that are "real" and that retain their "whole" form (meaning, they not been refined). Quinoa is a staple grain in the diet of the ancient Incas that you could cook up in about twenty minutes – this makes it easy for you to serve it as a quick side dish for busy weeknights. You can have your fill of fiber from barley, which is especially filling when paired with mushrooms in a rich, steamy soup. For cold winter mornings, go for a piping-hot bowl of breakfast oatmeal. Your favorite popcorn is also a type of whole grain; to keep it Mediterranean diet-friendly, skip the butter and just drizzle air-popped corn with olive oil.

You can consume whole wheat pasta, whole wheat bread, and other whole grain products to supplement your intake of whole grains. Just make sure to search the term "whole grain" or "whole" on the labels as well as in the in the list of ingredients, where it has to be the first ingredient. However, if switching from refined to whole grain proves difficult for you, you can introduce whole grain to your diet gradually by mixing one part whole grain with one part refined grain, or using whole-grain rice and pasta blends.

5. Amp up your protein intake.

Aim to replace most of the red meat in your diet with skinless turkey, skinless chicken and fish as well as plants like nuts and beans. This way, you get to reduce your intake of saturated fats. Another way of displacing red meat is to eat fish instead. Any kind of fish can be included in the Mediterranean diet as long as it not fried. You can eat fatty fish like tuna and salmon twice per week to benefit from their rich omega-3 fatty acid content, which is associated with improved cardiovascular health.

It helps to make vegetables and whole grains the stars of your meals, and to simply treat meat as a type of flavoring. When making pasta, for example, you can add a small handful of diced pancetta in the tomato sauce. But it is still alright to indulge in the occasional steak, as long as you settle for lean cuts such as sirloin, strip steak, flank steak and top loin. Remember to keep your portion size down to just three of four ounces.

6. Munch on seeds and nuts or low-fat cheese and other low-fat dairy products instead of snacking on unhealthy processed foods.

Ditch the usual processed foods like cookies and chips, which are loaded with sugars as well as trans fats and saturated fats. Instead, snack on sunflower seeds, walnuts or almonds (one handful). You can also enjoy eating non-fat/low-fat plain yogurt topped with fresh fruit or low-fat (calcium-rich) cheese as a healthy, portable snack.

7. Enjoy your food.

Make sure you have enough time to relish every bite of your Mediterranean diet foods. It also helps to treat the Mediterranean diet plan as a lifestyle that will help you lose weight and live longer. Avoid eating meals while watching television; you will be better off sitting down at the table and enjoying your meals at a leisurely pace with your family and friends. This will help you eat mindfully as you tune in to the signals of hunger and fullness that your body is giving out. You will find that you are more likely to eat until your hunger is satisfied than until you can hardly breathe from too much food.

8. Drink alcohol moderately.

If you can't give up alcohol, you have to make sure you are drinking it in moderate amounts (just one to two glasses) with a meal. As research has shown, moderate drinkers may be more likely to reduce their risk of heart disease than those who do not drink at all. This could be due to the fact that alcohol may play a role in raising the levels of good cholesterol in your body. In fact, wine has the ability to "thin" the blood or make it less likely to clot. Wine also contains antioxidants that help prevent the buildup of bad cholesterol in your arteries. It helps to keep in mind that one alcoholic drink equals five ounces of wine, one and a half ounces of liquor, or twelve ounces of beer.

Chapter 2 Week 1: Let's Do This!

DAY ONE

Breakfast

Heartwarming Egg and Toast

(266 calories)

- Bread, whole wheat, toasted (1 slice)
- Egg, large (1 piece) – cooked in olive oil (1/4 teaspoon) and seasoned with salt (a pinch) and pepper (a dash)
- Avocado, medium, mashed (1/4 piece)

Serve toast topped with egg and mashed avocado.

- Clementine (1 piece)

Morning Snack

Chickpeas

(131 calories)

- Hot and Spicy "Nuts" (1/4 cup) - Place rack in the oven's upper-third portion before setting the oven to 450 degrees to preheat. Blot-dry rinsed canned chickpeas (15 ounces) and then toss in a large bowl with olive oil (1 tablespoon), ground cumin (2 teaspoons), dried marjoram (1 teaspoon), ground allspice (1/4 teaspoon) and salt (1/4 teaspoon). Spread mixture on a baking sheet (rimmed) and place in the oven to bake for about twenty-five to thirty minutes or until the chickpeas are crunchy and browned. Let stand for about fifteen minutes to cool before serving.

Lunch

Gnocchi and Greens
(332 calories)

- Greens, mixed (2 cups) - topped with olive oil (1/2 tablespoon) and balsamic vinaigrette (1/2 tablespoon)
- Artichoke and Tomato Gnocchi (1 cup) - Heat a large skillet (nonstick) on medium-high before adding olive oil (1 tablespoon). Once oil is heated, add

gnocchi (16 ounces) and cook for five minutes or until plumped and lightly browned. Pour the cooked gnocchi into a large bowl and keep warm by covering. Meanwhile, lower heat to medium before adding olive oil (1 tablespoon) along with sliced onions (1 small piece). Cook for about two to three minutes or until lightly browned, then stir in diced red bell pepper (1 small piece). Cook for three minutes or until crisp-tender, then add thinly sliced garlic (4 large cloves) and chopped fresh oregano (1 tablespoon). Stir and cook for about thirty seconds before adding rinsed chickpeas (15 ounces), diced tomatoes (14 ounces) and chopped artichoke hearts (9 ounces). Stir well and cook for another three minutes before adding sliced pitted Kalamata olives (8 pieces), red wine vinegar (1 tablespoon) and the cooked gnocchi. Serve sprinkled with ground pepper (1/4 teaspoon).

Afternoon Snack

Fruit

(25 calories)

- Apricots, dried (3 pieces)

Dinner

Cherry Tomatoes with Couscous and Cod

(447 calories)

- Cherry tomatoes (1/2 cup) and sliced zucchini (1 cup) - sautéed in olive oil (1/2 tablespoon) and seasoned with pepper (a dash) and salt (a pinch)
- Cod (5 ounces) - cooked in olive oil (1 teaspoon) and seasoned with parsley or other herbs
- Pita round, whole wheat, toasted (1 six-and-one-half-inch piece)
- Lemon (1 wedge) as garnish

DAY TWO

Breakfast

Fruit with Cottage Cheese

(193 calories)

- Fresh fruit (1 piece) or canned fruit (1/2 cup)
- Cottage cheese, nonfat (2/3 cup)
- Almonds (6 pieces)

Serve cottage cheese topped with the nuts and fruits.

Morning Snack

Green Salad

(64 calories)

- Salad greens (1 cup)
- Balsamic vinaigrette (1 teaspoon) – combined with mixed herbs (1/2 teaspoon)

Toss greens and vinaigrette before serving.

Lunch

Hummus Sandwich

(298 calories)

- Hummus (1/3 cup)
- Milk, nonfat (1 cup)
- Cucumber slices (1/2 cup)
- Tomatoes (1/2 cup)
- Pita, whole wheat (1/2 piece)
- Lettuce, sliced (1/2 cup)

Spread the inside of pita with hummus before stuffing with lettuce, tomato and cucumber. Enjoy with milk.

Afternoon Snack

Orange Smoothie

(158 calories)

- Orange (1 piece)
- Ice (2 cups)
- Vanilla extract (1 teaspoon)
- Milk, nonfat (4 cup)

Process ingredients in the blender until smooth, then serve.

Dinner

Roasted Lamb with Couscous and Green Beans

(594 calories)

- Lamb chop (4 ounces) – basted with dressing and roasted at 450 degrees for ten minutes on both sides
- Dressing, lemon and herb (3 tablespoons)
- Green beans, fresh (1 cup) – steamed/microwaved until tender
- Couscous, cooked, w/out added oil (2/3 cup)

Serve couscous topped with the lamb chop and surrounded by the green beans.

DAY THREE

Breakfast

Oatmeal with Apple and Nuts

(297 calories)

- Oatmeal (1/2 cup) – cooked in water (1/2 cup) and skim milk (1/2 cup)
- Apple, medium, sliced (1/2 piece)

- Walnuts, chopped (1 tablespoon)

Serve oatmeal topped with walnuts, apple and cinnamon (a pinch).

Morning Snack

Fruit

(47 calories)

- Apple, medium (1/2 piece)

Lunch

Spicy Green Salad

(320 calories)

- Greens, mixed (2 cups)
- Cucumber slices (1/2 cup)
- Cherry tomatoes, halved (5 pieces)
- Feta cheese (1 tablespoon)
- Kalamata olives, pitted (5 pieces)
- Hot and Spicy "Nuts" (1/4 cup) – see Day One: Morning Snack for directions in making

Mix everything well. Serve salad topped with olive oil (1/2 tablespoon) and balsamic vinaigrette (1/2 tablespoon).

Afternoon Snack

Fruit

(51 calories)

- Apricots, dried (6 pieces)

Dinner

Roasted Salmon

(457 calories)

- Salmon fillet, roasted (5 ounces) – coated with dried oregano (1/4 teaspoon) and olive oil (1/4 teaspoon), then seasoned with salt (a pinch) and pepper (a dash)
- Fennel bulb, roasted (1 cup) – tossed with olive oil (1/2 tablespoon), pepper (a dash) and salt (a pinch)

- Couscous, whole wheat, cooked (1 cup) – topped with walnuts, chopped (1 tablespoon)
- Lemon (1 wedge) as garnish

DAY FOUR

Breakfast

Toast and Banana

(279 calories)

- Toast, whole wheat (1 slice)
- Peanut butter (1 tablespoon)
- Banana, medium (1 piece)

Morning Snack

Nuts

(65 calories)

- Walnuts (5 halves)

Lunch

Salad Greens and Hummus with Pita Bread

(350 calories)

- Greens, mixed (2 cups)
- Cucumber, sliced (1/2 cup)
- Carrot, grated (2 tablespoons)

Serve salad topped with balsamic vinegar (1/2 tablespoon) and olive oil (1/2 tablespoon). Enjoy with 6 1/2 -inch toasted pita round (whole wheat) and hummus (3 tablespoons) for dipping.

Afternoon Snack

Yogurt and Fruit

(80 calories)

- Greek yogurt, plain, nonfat (1/2 cup)
- Strawberries, sliced (1/4 cup)

Enjoy yogurt topped with strawberries.

Dinner

Savory Egg Drop Soup with Arugula and Toast

(416 calories)

- Arugula (2 cups) – topped with balsamic vinegar (1/2 tablespoon) and olive oil (1/2 tablespoon)
- Bread, whole wheat, toasted (1 slice) – drizzled with olive oil (1 teaspoon)
- Savory Egg Drop Soup (1 ½ cups) – Mix chicken broth (6 cups), freshly grated nutmeg (a pinch), scallion whites (1/2 bunch), small pasta (1 1/3 cups), rinsed chickpeas (7 ounces), and water (2 cups) in the Dutch oven. Cook covered on high until boiling. Remove cover and boil for three to five minutes more. Add chopped arugula (3 cups) and stir well. Cook for one minute or until wilted, then lower heat to medium-low. Keep stirring the soup as you gradually add lightly beaten eggs (4 large pieces), then cook for about two minutes or until the cooked egg appears like feathery strands. Add pepper and salt to season the soup before adding scallion greens

(1/2 bunch) as well. Serve in 5 bowls topped with Parmesan cheese.

DAY FIVE

Breakfast

Fruity and Nutty Oatmeal

(276 calories)

- Oatmeal (1/2 cup) – cooked in skim milk (1/2 cup) and water (1/2 cup)
- Walnuts, chopped (1 tablespoon)
- Strawberries, sliced (1/2 cup)

Sprinkle oatmeal with cinnamon (a pinch) before serving with walnuts and strawberries.

Morning Snack

Fruit

(70 calories)

- Clementines (2 pieces)

Lunch

Salad Greens with Hot and Spicy "Nuts"

(320 calories)

- Hot and Spicy "Nuts" (1/4 cup) – see Day One: Morning Snack for directions in making
- Greens, mixed (2 cups)
- Cherry tomatoes, halved (5 pieces)
- Feta cheese (1 tablespoon)
- Cucumber slices (1/2 cup)
- Kalamata olives, pitted (5 pieces)

Combine "nuts", greens, cherry tomatoes, cheese, cucumber and olives. Top with olive oil (1/2 tablespoon) and balsamic vinaigrette (1/2 tablespoon).

Afternoon Snack

Nuts and fruit

(108 calories)

- Walnuts, halved (5 pieces)
- Apricots, dried (5 pieces)

Dinner

Yummy Leftovers

(427 calories)

- Artichoke and Tomato Gnocchi (1 ¾ cups) – see Day One: Lunch for directions in making

Chapter 3 Week 2: We're Getting There!

DAY SIX

Breakfast

Egg and Toast with Avocado

(266 calories)

- Bread, whole wheat, toasted (1 slice)
- Avocado, medium, mashed (1/4 piece)
- Egg, large (1 piece) – cooked in olive oil (1/4 teaspoon) and seasoned with pepper (a dash) and salt (a pinch)

Serve toast topped with egg and avocado alongside clementines (2 small pieces).

Morning Snack

Fruit

(95 calories)

- Apple, medium (1 piece)

Lunch

Pita Bread and Salad Greens

(350 calories)

- Greens, mixed (2 cups)
- Cucumber, sliced (1/2 cup)
- Carrot, grated (2 tablespoons)
- Pita round, whole wheat, toasted (1 6 ½-inch piece)
- Hummus (3 tablespoon) as dipping
- Olive oil (1/2 tablespoon)
- Balsamic vinegar (1/2 tablespoon)

Serve salad topped with balsamic vinegar and olive oil, alongside the toasted pita and hummus.

Afternoon Snack

Fruit

(27 calories)

- Strawberries, sliced (1/4 cup)

Dinner

Tasty Tuna Salad

(444 calories)

- Bread, whole wheat, toasted (1 slice)
- Tasty Tuna Salad (1 serving) – Combine water (1 ½ tablespoons), lemon juice (1 ½ tablespoons) and tahini (1 ½ tablespoons) in a large mixing bowl. Stir in chopped and pitted Kalamata olives (4 pieces), parsley (2 tablespoons), drained light tuna (5 ounces) and feta cheese (2

tablespoons). Mix well.

Serve tuna salad on top of baby spinach (2 cups) alongside a peeled orange (1 medium piece).

DAY SEVEN

Breakfast

Apple and Cinnamon Oatmeal

(297 calories)

- Oatmeal (1/2 cup) – cooked in water (1/2 cup) and skim milk (1/2 cup)
- Apple, diced (1/2 piece)
- Walnuts, chopped (1 tablespoon)

Serve chopped walnuts and diced apple on top of cooked oatmeal. Add cinnamon (a pinch) and enjoy.

Morning Snack

Fruit

(152 calories)

- Apple, medium (1/2 piece)
- Peanut butter (1 tablespoon)

Lunch

Yummy Leftovers

(305 calories)

- Arugula (2 cups) mixed with balsamic vinegar (1/2 tablespoon) and olive oil (1/2 tablespoon)
- Savory Egg Drop Soup (1 ½ cups) – see Day Four: Dinner for directions in making

Afternoon Snack

Fruit

(27 calories)

- Strawberries, sliced (1/2 cup)

Dinner

Roast Pork with Cherry Tomatoes and Asparagus

(400 calories)

- Roast Pork with Cherry Tomatoes and Asparagus (1 serving) – Set the oven to 400 degrees to preheat. Fill a medium saucepan (heated on medium-high) with 2 ½ cups of water and bring to a boil. After removing from heat, add bulgur (1 ¼ cups) and salt (1/4 teaspoon) and stir well. Let stand, covered, for about twenty minutes or until tender. In the meantime, stir together salt (1/4 teaspoon), dried marjoram (1 teaspoon), and ground pepper (1/4 teaspoon) in a small bowl. Once combined, sprinkle on the trimmed pork tenderloin (1 pound). Heat a large ovenproof or cast-iron skillet on medium-high before adding canola oil (1 tablespoon). Place seasoned pork tenderloin on top of heated oil and, turning several times, cook for about four to six minutes or until browned. Place one-inch trimmed asparagus cubes (1 bunch) in a mixing bowl and mix along with chopped red onion (1 large piece), canola oil (1 tablespoon), and salt (1/4 teaspoon). Scatter the asparagus-onion mixture around the browned pork before transferring to the oven. Roast for about twelve to sixteen minutes or until the thermometer registers 145 degrees. When the pork is just about to be done, add halved cherry tomatoes (1 cup) to the bowl with the asparagus-onion mixture. Transfer the cooked pork onto a large cutting board; let sit for about five minutes and then slice. Meanwhile, add the mixed vegetables to the pan juices and toss well. After draining any liquid left in the bulgur, add lemon juice (2 tablespoons), lemon zest (2 teaspoons), and chopped fresh parsley (1/2 cup) and stir well. In a mixing bowl, combine plain hummus (1/4 cup) with hot water (2 tablespoons). Arrange the prepared bulgur in four bowls. Serve topped with the vegetables and pork and drizzled with hummus sauce.

DAY EIGHT

Breakfast

Whole Wheat Toast

(279 calories)

- Toast, whole wheat (1 slice)
- Peanut butter (1 tablespoon)
- Banana, medium (1 piece)

Morning Snack

Easy Egg

(78 calories)

- Egg, hard-boiled (1 piece) — seasoned with salt (a pinch) and pepper (a dash)

Lunch

Hummus and Pita Bread with Green Salad

(299 calories)

- Feta cheese (1 tablespoon)
- Cucumber slices (1/2 cup)

- Cherry tomatoes, halved (5 pieces)
- Mixed greens (2 cups)

Mix feta cheese, cucumber slices, halved cherry tomatoes and mixed greens. Toss with a mixture of olive oil (1/2 tablespoon) and balsamic vinegar (1/2 tablespoon). Serve together with hummus dip (3 tablespoons) and toasted whole wheat pita (6 ½-inch round).

Afternoon Snack

Fruit

(95 calories)

- Apple, medium (1 piece)

Dinner

Prosciutto-wrapped Chicken with Toasted Couscous and Steamed Broccoli

(484 calories)

- Couscous, whole wheat, toasted (1/2

cup)
- Broccoli florets, steamed (1 cup)
- Prosciutto-wrapped Chicken (1 serving) – Between layers of plastic wrap, place skinless, boneless, and with-tenders-removed chicken breasts (2 five-ounce pieces). Use a meat mallet's smooth side or a rolling pin to bash the chicken breasts to about a quarter-inch thickness without breaking them up. Sprinkle round pepper (1/4 teaspoon) on the chicken slices to season and wrap each with a thinly sliced prosciutto. Top each prosciutto-wrapped chicken with one to two sage leaves before dusting all-purpose flour (1 ½ teaspoons) on both sides. Meanwhile, heat a large skillet on medium before adding butter (1 tablespoon) and olive oil (2 teaspoons). Add the chicken and cook for three minutes on each side or until no pink meat shows in the center. Once done (any juice running out from the meat should be without a trace of pink color), place the chicken on a warm platter and then let sit covered with foil.

Pour dry Marsala (3/4 cup) in the pan and cook on high for three to four minutes or until thickened and reduced to half its original volume. Serve chicken topped with the Marsala sauce and enjoy with toasted couscous and steamed broccoli florets.

DAY NINE

Breakfast

Heavenly Yogurt Parfait

(280 calories)

- Bran cereal (1/2 cup)
- Greek yogurt, nonfat, plain (6 ounces)
- Apricots, dried, sliced into small bits (4 pieces)
- Almonds, chopped (6 pieces) or nuts, roasted, chopped (1/4 cup)

Fill a tall glass with alternating layers of yogurt, apricots and bran cereal before topping with chopped almonds or roasted nuts.

Morning Snack

Fruit

(81 calories)

- Apple (1 piece)

Lunch

Hearty Lentil Soup

(250 calories)

- Olive oil (2 tablespoons)
- Onions, chopped (1/4 cup)
- Broth, vegetable/chicken (8 cups)
- Carrot, peeled, chopped (1 piece)
- Lentils, red (1 ½ cups)
- Pepper (1/2 teaspoon)

Heat a soup pot on medium before adding olive oil. Stir in onions and carrots; cook for five minutes or until tender. After rinsing the lentils, add to the onions and carrots. Stir in broth and allow the mixture to boil before reducing heat to low. Cover the soup pot halfway and allow mixture to simmer for thirty minutes or until the lentils are softened. Arrange your hearty lentil soup among six bowls and enjoy.

Afternoon Snack

Lemony Herbed Salad

(64 calories)

- Salad greens (1 cup)
- Dressing, lemon-and-herb or vinaigrette (1 tablespoon)

Enjoy salad greens after tossing with the dressing.

Dinner

Shrimp Kebabs with Steamed Veggies and Basmati Rice

(629 calories)

- Vegetables, mixed, fresh/frozen (1 cup) – steamed

- Margarine (1 teaspoon)
- Grape tomatoes (4 pieces)
- Shrimp, peeled, deveined (4 ounces)
- Dressing/marinade, lemon and herb (4 tablespoons)
- Basmati rice, cooked (2/3 cup)
- Mushrooms, whole (4 pieces)
- Onions, thickly sliced (4 one-inch pieces)

In a large bowl, combine shrimp with the onions, tomatoes, mushrooms and dressing. Place one of each on skewers and bake in the preheated oven (500 degrees) for fifteen minutes. Serve shrimp kebabs on top of basmati rice surrounded with steamed vegetables.

DAY TEN

Breakfast

Yogurt and Cheese

(190 calories)

- Cottage cheese, nonfat (1/4 cup)
- Honey (1 tablespoon)

- Greek/plain yogurt, nonfat (6 ounces)

Serve cottage cheese topped with a mixture of the yogurt and honey.

Morning Snack

Mixed Berries Smoothie

(120 calories)

- Milk, nonfat (1 cup)
- Sugar substitute (1 packer)
- Mixed berries, frozen (3/4 cup)
- Ice (2 cups)

Fill a blender with the ice. Add nonfat milk, sugar substitute and frozen mixed berries and process until smooth.

Lunch

Fig and Spinach Salad

(565 calories)

- Walnut halves (4 pieces)
- Grape tomatoes (5 pieces)

- Baby spinach, raw (3 cups)
- Chickpeas, drained, rinsed (1/2 cup)
- Cucumber, sliced (1 piece)
- Vinaigrette, light (4 tablespoons)
- Turkish figs, organic, sliced (2 pieces)

Toss walnuts, grape tomatoes, chickpeas, cucumber, figs and spinach with the vinaigrette.

Afternoon Snack

Banana Shake

(143 calories)

- Greek/plain yogurt, nonfat (1/3 cup)
- Banana (1 piece)
- Sugar substitute (1 packet)
- Milk, nonfat (1/2 cup)
- Ice (2 cups)

Fill a blender with the yogurt, banana, sugar substitute, milk, and ice. Process until smooth and enjoy.

Dinner

Chicken Kebabs with Spinach and Basmati Rice

(596 calories)

- Basmati rice, cooked (2/3 cup) – cook according to package directions without any added fat; once cooked, add margarine (2 teaspoons) on top and allow to melt in.
- Spinach, steamed (2 cups) – Place fresh spinach in a covered pot (don't add any water) and steam until spinach is cooked.
- Chicken kebabs (1 serving) – Slice chicken breast (4 ounces) into one-inch cubes then baste with lemon-and-herb marinade (4 tablespoons). Arrange basted chicken cubes on skewer along with mushrooms (4 small pieces), onion (4 one-inch pieces), and grape tomatoes (4 pieces). Place in the oven to bake for about five minutes.

Chapter 4 Tips and Tricks for Preparing Meals the Mediterranean Way

Following the Mediterranean Diet plan to lose weight effectively and live longer is easier when you have these tips and tricks to help you along.

Vegetables

1. Grilled vegetables are always a treat, but you can also buy frozen vegetables and place them in the microwave for two to three minutes. Make sure to use a container that is microwave-safe and cover with plastic wrap.

2. You can make use of bagged salad mixes for convenience.

Grains

1. Use couscous as part of your Mediterranean diet plan. It cooks very quickly and can even be interchanged with basmati rice and other grains that take longer to cook.

2. For those days when you have no time to spare for complicated meals, stock up on instant brown rice that you can just boil straight in the bag. Cook for just ten minutes and it's good to eat.

3. Whole wheat pita is a great replacement for rice, beans, couscous and pasta in recipes that call for starch.

Meats

1. Take advantage of frozen grilled fish – it can be a healthy replacement for any fish included in the Mediterranean diet plan.

2. For salad recipes that require grilled chicken, you can make use of deli slice turkey or chicken.

3. Purchase salmon and tuna burgers; you can find them in the grocery's freezer section. You can simply bake or grill them up to replace other kinds of Mediterranean diet-friendly fish.

4. You may also use pre-grilled chicken to make your meals meatier.

5. Packaged tuna and canned salmon may also be used as healthy ingredients in the Mediterranean diet.

Others

1. Simplicity is key to eating the Mediterranean way. The Mediterranean diet plan is all about preparing healthy ingredients in simple ways to ensure bringing out the food's flavors. As much as possible, use fresh and wholesome ingredients; say no to processed foods. As the meals in the Mediterranean diet plan do not really take that long to prepare, you are left with more time to enjoy eating them.

2. You can always double or even triple your recipe ingredients, especially if you do not mind eating leftovers. This way, you can either make your meals last for a couple of days, or store them in plastic containers and freeze (simply reheat in the microwave).

3. Try growing and cultivating a vegetable or herb garden in your backyard. You will enjoy harvesting your own edible garden, and you can always swap produce with your neighbors.

4. To save time, make sure to stock up on olive oil and other pantry staples such as jarred tomatoes, pasta, whole grains and olives. You can then simply pick up fresh ingredients from the store a few times per week.

5. Throw away your salt shaker. You can add taste and flair to your meals with the help of citrus and herbs. Bring your meals to life with rosemary, basil, garlic, mint, oregano, lemon, thyme and mint.

Conclusion

It is my sincere hope that you might have liked all the recipes which have been mentioned in the book and once again thank you for getting this book and experimenting with the recipes.

About The Author

Avent Lavoie is born with the vision to promote *Mediterranean diet* among the masses. The author has written several research papers on the topic. He has served as an instructor promoting various cultural arts in University of San Francisco. He is currently living with his spouse in Texas.

www.ingramcontent.com/pod-product-compliance
Lightning Source LLC
LaVergne TN
LVHW021048100526
838202LV00079B/4881